I0774113

Table of Contents

INTTRODUCTION

The specific carbohydrate (SCD) diet is an increasingly popular dietary approach that restricts foods high in carbohydrates to promote weight loss, improve gut health, and aid overall digestive health. It was first developed many decades ago for the management of celiac disease. However, it is now being considered and studied for use in other conditions, such as Crohn's disease and ulcerative colitis (two types of inflammatory bowel disease, or IBD). This book provides a comprehensive beginner's guide to the SCD diet and a meal plan based on this approach.

CHAPTER ONE

Overview

The Specific Carbohydrate Diet, known as the SCD Diet, has a large cult following among individuals with inflammatory bowel diseases (IBD). Learn more about what it is, what foods are acceptable, and what the research says.

What is the Specific Carbohydrate Diet?

SCD is an elimination diet that emphasizes removing certain types of carbohydrate-containing foods based on their chemical structure. The governing theory behind SCD is that complex carbs encourage an overgrowth of unhealthy bacteria in your small intestine if you have IBD. As these bacteria grow, they produce byproducts that promote inflammation and eventually lead to reduced absorption of nutrients in your digestive tract. SCD proponents claim that it inhibits the growth of such bacteria and restores digestive function by eliminating all carbohydrate food sources with two or more linked sugar molecules. Though many carbs are prohibited, the SCD does permit carb sources that have single, unbound sugar molecules — or monosaccharides — as your digestive tract absorbs them more easily.

What are the concepts behind the Specific Carbohydrate Diet?

Carbohydrates have significant potential to influence the health of the microbiome. In IBD, undigested carbohydrates in the GI tract, particularly complex carbohydrates, starches, and lactose, can become excessively fermented by pathogenic intestinal bacteria. This leads to overgrowth of these bad bacteria, which cause inflammation and injury to the mucosal lining of the gut. The SCD Diet is centered around the concept that foods which contain one sugar molecule (such as glucose) are more readily digested and absorbed, which will halt the overpopulation of bad bacteria, allow the gut to heal, and improve the balance of the gut microorganisms. Along with the more easily digested carbs, the SCD Diet includes probiotics in the form of yogurt which has been fermented for 24 hours to eliminate the lactose.

Do I lose weight on the Specific Carbohydrate Diet?

The SCD is not a weight loss program, contrary to popular belief. Because the SCD diet is so restricted and lacks evidence of efficacy, patients suffering from gastrointestinal issues may prefer to try other diets such as the low FODMAP diet or a gluten-free diet.

How does the Specific Carbohydrate Diet work?

The theory behind the SCD is to eliminate complex carbohydrates from the diet. However, simple carbohydrates are still allowed. The digestive system contains many different types of bacteria (which are part of the gut microbiome). Keeping them in balance is important because some types can cause symptoms if they grow too numerous. The theory of the SCD is that complex carbohydrates become food for potentially harmful bacteria. Therefore, avoiding certain carbohydrates may starve the harmful bacteria and allow beneficial types to flourish. Other food types avoided on the SCD include processed foods, food additives, preservatives, and sugar. Some of these types of foods have been shown to contribute to inflammation. It's thought that avoiding these foods might also help with symptoms within the digestive tract. Simple carbohydrates, which are easier to digest, are allowed on the SCD. The SCD is an eating plan with several progressive steps leading to a maintenance phase. It is meant to be used long-term to control symptoms. In some cases, people may introduce certain disallowed foods back into their diet on a limited basis upon reaching a year without symptoms.

What foods do I avoid with the Specific Carbohydrate Diet?

The diet labels any food or additive containing two or more chemically linked sugar molecules "illegal." The SCD guidebook, "Breaking the Vicious Cycle," collectively refers to these foods as complex carbs. In scientific terms, any food with disaccharides, oligosaccharides, or polysaccharides will appear on the list of illegal foods. As you can imagine, the list of banned foods is extensive. Common examples include:

• Potatoes

• Grains and pseudo-grains, including rice, wheat, corn, quinoa, and millet

• Processed meats and meats with additives

• Most dairy

• Most legumes

• Most processed sugar, artificial sweeteners, and sugar alcohols

The general structure of SCD is very rigid and intended to be followed exactly as outlined in the guidebook — with little to no room for flexibility. While some people may reintroduce certain banned foods after symptoms subside, this will vary depending on your response to the diet.

What foods do I eat with the Specific Carbohydrate Diet?

SCD-approved foods are collectively called "legal." Most of the foods on this list are unprocessed, whole foods that don't offer many complex carbs. The main sources of approved or "legal" carbs in the SCD come from the monosaccharides glucose, fructose, and galactose.

• Fruits: Most fresh or frozen fruits and juices. Canned fruits may be allowed if they don't have added sugar or starch.

• Vegetables: Most vegetables, except for potatoes, yams, plantains, and some other high-starch vegetables

• Meat: Most fresh meats, as long as they don't contain any fillers or additives

• Eggs

• Some dairy: Homemade yogurt fermented for at least 24 hours and some natural cheeses

• Certain legumes: Some dried legumes, as long as they're soaked and prepared according to the directions outlined in the guidebook

• Nuts and nut butter: Most nuts, as long as they're free from added starch or sugar

• Herbs and spices: Most dried or fresh herbs and spices. Prepackaged blends may contain additives and are typically discouraged

The SCD guidebook recommends eating only the explicitly legal foods to avoid inadvertently ingesting something banned.

Can the Specific Carbohydrate Diet be used to treat digestive disorders?

SCD was originally designed as a therapy for people with celiac disease and IBD, an umbrella term that includes ulcerative colitis and Crohn's disease. These diseases can hamper your ability to digest and absorb nutrients from food. Thus, SCD aims to heal intestinal tissue in order to restore its functions. SCD's promoters claim that some people are less adept at digesting foods — such as grains, legumes, refined sugar, and high-starch food additives — that result from settled agricultural practices and the modern food industry. Supporters assert that continued ingestion of these carbs leads to an overgrowth of unhealthy bacteria in your gut, which promotes inflammation and eventually diminishes your ability to digest. Strict adherence to SCD will purportedly starve these bacteria by depriving them of food, allowing your gut tissue to heal. To this day, SCD is primarily used to treat intestinal disorders — but with varied success. One of the major criticisms of this diet is its lack of concrete scientific evidence. Most available data is weak and limited to very small studies or anecdotal evidence, which isn't enough to state whether or not the SCD works definitively. Ultimately, more research is needed to determine whether SCD is truly an effective treatment for IBD.

Can the Specific Carbohydrate Diet be used for other medical conditions?

SCD is also marketed for people with other medical conditions, including autism spectrum disorder (ASD) and cystic fibrosis (CF). Early research suggests that gut bacteria may be crucial in treating some behavioral and inflammatory conditions, such as CF and ASD. SCD is believed to balance your digestive tract, leading its proponents to theorize that it may be an effective therapy for these conditions, too. However, the scientific understanding of these disorders is limited. Beyond anecdotal reports, there is no research to suggest that SCD treats diseases outside of IBD — if that. In fact, it's still unclear whether the SCD impacts gut bacteria at all. More research is needed to understand if SCD affects ASD or CF.

What are the health benefits of the Specific Carbohydrate Diet?

Some of the top health benefits of the SCD diet include better sleep, reduced inflammation, improved digestive health, improved overall health, and remission of symptoms of several digestive diseases.

• Better Sleep: Eating meals with fewer carbohydrates can help reduce nighttime restlessness, which may lead to better quality sleep.

• Reduced Inflammation: Restricting complex carbs in the diet can reduce inflammation, which is a primary factor in many chronic diseases.

• Improved Digestive Health: Eliminating complex carbs and eating more nutrient-dense, unprocessed foods can improve digestive health and reduce symptoms of digestive disorders.

• Improved Overall Health: Eating a diet full of nutrient-dense and unprocessed foods can help improve overall health.

• Remission of Symptoms of Several Digestive Diseases: Several studies have suggested that following the SCD diet can reduce symptoms associated with inflammatory conditions such as Crohn's disease and ulcerative colitis.

What are the health risks of the Specific Carbohydrate Diet?

Although the SCD diet benefits many people, some critical health concerns are possible with this diet such as malnutrition, increased bloating and weight loss.

• Malnutrition: The SCD diet restricts several food groups, which can lead to a lack of essential vitamins and minerals. Therefore, it is crucial to supplement your meals with multivitamins and other nutrient-dense foods.

• Increased Bloating: The SCD diet eliminates several food groups and can cause increased bloating. Therefore, it is crucial to monitor your digestion and adjust portions accordingly.

• Weight Loss: One of the unintended consequences of SCD is weight loss. Since the diet is so restrictive, some followers lose weight as they adjust their diet.

Who should do the Specific Carbohydrate Diet?

The SCD diet is best for people who want to improve their digestive health, including those with gastrointestinal diseases such as Crohn's disease and ulcerative colitis. It is important to note that you should not undertake the SCD diet without medical supervision as it can have serious side effects if followed incorrectly. Additionally, this diet is best for those who are generally healthy and looking to improve their overall health by eating nutritious, whole foods. While there is not a specific SCD bodybuilding diet, weightlifters and bodybuilders with digestive health problems can also follow the diet. The SCD bodybuilding diet can protect your digestive health while giving you ample lean protein to maximize your gains.

Is the Specific Carbohydrate Diet Right For Me?

The SCD Diet may be a helpful starting place, especially if it helps relieve symptoms of IBD. It may be a diet that is useful to temporarily get flares or other symptoms of IBD under control. Some people with IBD may benefit from a modified version of the SCD Diet that allows for more food options such as oats, rice, or soy. Following a flare, it is best to incorporate new foods gradually, as tolerated, to help you get adequate nutrition from your diet. Every person with IBD is unique and has different responses to different foods. Because of this, there is no single, uniform diet that is prescribed for IBD patients and the SCD Diet may not be feasible for everyone with Crohn's Disease or ulcerative colitis.

How easy is the Specific Carbohydrate Diet Program to Follow?

The SCD program is not easy to follow because it is extremely restrictive. Restaurants use many ingredients you are not allowed to eat. Additionally, the SCD program requires a lot of meal planning and preparation to ensure that all meals are SCD-friendly. It is essential to have the discipline to follow the SCD diet properly.

Before beginning the SCD, it's recommended that people who are experiencing severe symptoms, such as severe cramping and diarrhea, follow an introductory diet for two to five days before moving on to the SCD. During the introduction period, food intake is limited to just a few, easily digested foods. After completing two to five days of the introduction diet, you can start introducing SCD "legal" foods. There is no specified schedule for introducing SCD-legal foods, but there are certain guidelines that should be followed, including:

• Ripe fruits and vegetables should initially be peeled and cooked thoroughly.

• Most raw fruits and vegetables should not be introduced to the diet until diarrhea has subsided or is under control. Very ripe bananas with brown spots are the one exception to this rule.

• Slowly introduce new foods based on your symptoms.

• If foods seem to trigger or worsen symptoms such as gas or diarrhea when they are introduced, these foods should be removed and then reintroduced at a later time.

• SCD-legal foods that have caused symptoms in the past should be removed from the diet if they continue to cause symptoms after a week of elimination.

• Foods that contain carbohydrates other than those found in SCD-legal foods, such as fruits, honey, and SCD yogurt, are strictly forbidden.

The 7-Day Diet Plan

All grains are off-limits on this plan, including those that do not contain gluten. Fruits, both fresh and dried with no added sugar, and low-starch vegetables are allowed. Certain fruit juices with no added sugar, such as fresh-squeezed orange juice, are also acceptable. Meanwhile, most nuts are approved, but seeds are not. Lean protein sources—including meat, fish, and eggs—are permitted, as long as they are unprocessed with no additives. Some milk-derived dairy products are also included. Almost all added sugars and artificial sweeteners are banned. A week's food intake could look like the following:

• Day 1: Unlimited fresh fruit with a cup of coffee; salad with a side of asparagus; lentil salad

• Day 2: Unlimited fresh fruit with a cup of coffee; homemade plain yogurt with berries and honey; grilled eggplant with fresh fish

• Day 3: Unlimited fresh fruit with a cup of coffee; salad topped with nuts; sharp cheddar cheese slices and dairy-free tomato soup with no added sugar

• Day 4: Unlimited fresh fruit with a cup of coffee; salad with eggs and a handful of unsweetened dried fruits; dry curd unsweetened cottage cheese with grilled chicken

• Day 5: Unlimited fresh fruit with a cup of coffee; shrimp sautéed in oil and artichoke hearts

• Day 6: Unlimited fresh fruit with a cup of coffee; green bean salad topped with cheddar cheese; two boiled eggs and salmon filet cooked in olive oil

• Day 7: Unlimited fresh fruit with a cup of coffee; unsweetened juice with boiled eggs and a slice of Swiss cheese; a handful of raw cashews; grilled fish of your choice and a side of mushrooms sauteed in oil.

CHAPTER TWO

Specific Carbohydrate Diet Recipes

Mongolian Strawberry Orange Juice Smoothie

Prep Time: 10 mins

Total Time: 10 mins

Servings: 4

Ingredients

• 1 cup chopped fresh strawberries

• 1 cup orange juice

• 10 cubes ice

- 1 tablespoon sugar

Directions

1. In a blender, combine strawberries, orange juice, ice cubes, and sugar. Blend until smooth. Pour into glasses and serve.

Nutrition Facts (per serving)

52 Calories

0g Fat

13g Carbs

1g Protein

Pinto Beans With Mexican-Style Seasonings

Prep Time: 15 mins

Servings: 8

Ingredients

- 1 pound dried pinto beans, rinsed

- 4 cups water, or as needed

• 2 (10 ounce) cans diced tomatoes with green chile peppers (such as RO*TEL®)

• ½ pound bacon, cut into 1/2-inch pieces

• 1 yellow onion, chopped

• 1 tablespoon chili powder, or to taste

• 1 tablespoon ground cumin, or to taste

• 1 ½ teaspoons garlic powder, or to taste

• ½ bunch fresh cilantro, chopped

• salt to taste

Directions

1. Place pinto beans into a large pot and pour in enough water to cover by 2 to 3 inches. Let beans soak overnight.

2. Drain beans, return to pot, and pour in fresh water to cover; add tomatoes, bacon, onion, chili powder, cumin, and garlic powder. Bring to a boil, reduce heat to low, and simmer for 3 hours. Check the beans occasionally and add more water if needed.

3. Stir cilantro and salt into beans simmer until beans are soft, about 1 more hour.

Nutrition Facts (per serving)

267 Calories

5g Fat

41g Carbs

16g Protein

Amazing Lentils and Kale

Prep Time: 15 mins

Cook Time: 55 mins

Total Time: 1 hr 10 mins

Servings: 6

Yield: 6 servings

Ingredients

• 2 tablespoons olive oil

• 1 cup shredded carrot

- 1 cup chopped onion

- 5 cloves garlic, minced

- 6 cups vegetable broth

- 1 (16 ounce) package dry lentils

- 1 (24 ounce) jar chunky-style salsa

- 1 pinch cayenne pepper, or to taste

- salt and ground black pepper to taste

- 1 bunch kale, chopped

Directions

1. Heat olive oil in a large pot over medium heat. Cook and stir shredded carrot, chopped onion, and minced garlic in the hot oil until softened, 5 to 7 minutes.

2. Pour vegetable broth into the pot. Stir lentils and salsa into the broth mixture. Bring to a boil, place a cover on the pot, and cook at a simmer until the lentils are softened, about 45 minutes.

3. Season the lentil mixture with cayenne pepper, salt, and black pepper.

4. Stir kale into the lentil mixture. Replace the cover onto the pot and cook just until the kale is wilted, 3 to 5 minutes.

Cook's Note:

Use chicken broth in place of vegetable broth if you prefer.

Tip

Aluminum foil helps keep food moist, ensures it cooks evenly, keeps leftovers fresh, and makes clean-up easy.

Nutrition Facts (per serving)

377 Calories

7g Fat

62g Carbs

23g Protein

These vegan black bean quesadillas pack a big punch, minus the fat of all that cheese! Serve with guacamole.

Prep Time: 10 mins

Cook Time: 45 mins

Total Time: 55 mins

Servings: 4

Yield: 4 quesadillas

Ingredients

• 1 (15 ounce) can great Northern beans, drained and rinsed

• 1 cup diced tomatoes, divided

• 1 clove garlic

• ⅓ cup nutritional yeast

• 1 teaspoon ground cumin

• ¼ teaspoon chili powder

• salt to taste

• 1 pinch cayenne pepper, or to taste

• ½ cup black beans, drained and rinsed

• 1 tablespoon olive oil, or as needed

• 8 whole grain tortillas

• cooking spray

Directions

1. Blend great Northern beans, 3/4 cup tomatoes, and garlic in a food processor until smooth. Add nutritional yeast, cumin, chili powder, salt, and cayenne pepper and blend until combined.

2. Transfer bean mixture to a large bowl. Stir in black beans and remaining 1/4 cup tomatoes.

3. Heat olive oil in a large skillet over medium-high heat. Place a tortilla in hot oil. Spread about 1/4 cup filling over tortilla. Place another tortilla on top of filling; cook until filling is warmed, about 10 minutes.

4. Spray the top tortilla with cooking spray and flip quesadilla to cook the second side until lightly browned,

3 to 5 minutes. Repeat with remaining tortillas and filling.

Nutrition Facts (per serving)

416 Calories

6g Fat

86g Carbs

23g Protein

Vegan Black Bean Burgers

Prep Time: 15 mins

Cook Time: 20 mins

Total Time: 35 mins

Servings: 4

Ingredients

• 1 (15 ounce) can black beans, drained and rinsed

• 3 baby carrots, grated (Optional)

• ⅓ cup chopped sweet onion

- ¼ cup minced green bell pepper (Optional)

- 1 tablespoon minced garlic

- 3 tablespoons chile-garlic sauce (such as Sriracha®), or to taste

- 1 tablespoon cornstarch

- 1 tablespoon warm water

- 1 teaspoon chili powder

- 1 teaspoon ground cumin

- 1 teaspoon seafood seasoning (such as Old Bay®)

- ¼ teaspoon salt

- ¼ teaspoon ground black pepper

- 2 slices whole-wheat bread, torn into small crumbs

- ¾ cup unbleached flour, or as needed

Directions

1. Preheat the oven to 350 degrees F (175 degrees C). Grease a baking sheet.

2. Mash black beans in a bowl. Add carrots, onion, bell pepper, and garlic; mix well.

3. Whisk chile-garlic sauce, cornstarch, water, chili powder, cumin, seafood seasoning, salt, and black pepper together in a separate small bowl.

4. Stir chile-garlic sauce mixture into black bean mixture; mix in bread crumbs. Stir flour, 1/4 cup at a time, into bean mixture until a sticky batter forms.

5. Spoon mounds of batter onto the prepared baking sheet, about a 3/4-inch thickness per mound; shape into burgers.

6. Bake in the preheated oven until cooked in the center and crisp on the outside, about 10 minutes per side.

Recipe Tip

One egg can be substituted for cornstarch, but the recipe will not be vegan.

Nutrition Facts (per serving)

264 Calories

1g Fat

52g Carbs

12g Protein

Copycat Panera Broccoli Cheddar Soup

Prep Time: 15 mins

Cook Time: 45 mins

Total Time: 1 hr

Servings: 8

Ingredients

- 1 tablespoon butter

- ½ onion, chopped

- ¼ cup melted butter

- ¼ cup flour

- 2 cups milk

- 2 cups chicken stock

- 1 ½ cups coarsely chopped broccoli florets

- 1 cup matchstick-cut carrots

- 1 stalk celery, thinly sliced

- 2 ½ cups shredded sharp Cheddar cheese

- salt and ground black pepper to taste

Directions

1. Melt 1 tablespoon butter in a skillet over medium-high heat. Add onion; cook and stir until tender and translucent, about 5 minutes. Set aside.

2. Whisk 1/4 cup melted butter and flour together in a large saucepan over medium-low heat. Continue to whisk and cook, adding 1 to 2 tablespoons of milk if necessary to keep the flour from burning, 3 to 4 minutes.

3. Gradually add milk while whisking constantly; stir in chicken stock and bring to a simmer. Cook until mixture is thickened, about 20 minutes. Add broccoli, carrots, celery, and sautéed onion; simmer until all the vegetables are tender, about 15 minutes.

4. Stir in Cheddar cheese until melted; season with salt and pepper to taste before serving.

Nutrition Facts (per serving)

304 Calories

23g Fat

11g Carbs

14g Protein

Lemon Chicken Orzo Soup

This lemon chicken orzo soup is comfort in a bowl. It is so flavorful with tender pieces of chicken in a lemony broth with orzo pasta, carrots, onions, celery, and baby spinach. This has quickly become one of my family's favorite soup recipes.

Prep Time: 20 mins

Cook Time: 30 mins

Total Time: 50 mins

Servings:12

Yield: 6 quarts

Ingredients

- 8 ounces orzo pasta

- 1 teaspoon olive oil

- 3 medium carrots, chopped, or more to taste

- 3 ribs celery, chopped

- 1 medium onion, chopped

- 2 cloves garlic, minced

- ½ teaspoon dried thyme

- ½ teaspoon dried oregano

- salt and ground black pepper to taste

- 1 bay leaf

- 3 (32 ounce) cartons fat-free, low-sodium chicken broth

- ½ cup fresh lemon juice

- 1 lemon, zested

- 8 ounces cooked chicken breast, chopped

- 1 (8 ounce) package baby spinach leaves

• 1 lemon, sliced for garnish (Optional)

• ¼ cup grated Parmesan cheese (Optional)

Directions

1. Bring a large pot of lightly salted water to a boil. Stir in orzo and return to a boil. Cook pasta uncovered until partially cooked through but not yet soft, about 5 minutes; drain and rinse with cold water until cooled completely.

2. Meanwhile, heat olive oil in a large pot over medium heat. Add carrots, celery, and onion; cook and stir until vegetables begin to soften and onion becomes translucent, about 5 minutes. Add garlic; cook and stir until fragrant, about 1 minute more. Season mixture with thyme, oregano, bay leaf, salt, and black pepper; continue cooking another 30 seconds before pouring chicken broth into the pot.

3. Bring broth to a boil. Partially cover the pot, reduce heat to medium-low, and simmer until vegetables are just tender, about 10 minutes.

4. Stir orzo, lemon juice, and lemon zest into broth; add chicken. Cook until chicken and orzo are heated through, about 5 minutes. Add baby spinach; cook until spinach wilts into broth and orzo is tender, 2 to 3 minutes. Ladle soup into bowls; garnish with lemon slices and Parmesan cheese.

Nutrition Facts (per serving)

167 Calories

4g Fat

22g Carbs

12g Protein

Greek Lemon Chicken Soup

This Greek lemon chicken soup is a perfect introduction to a full Greek meal or a hearty bowlful for a meal in itself. Serve with fresh pita triangles, and you'll be sure to please your guests!

Prep Time: 20 mins

Cook Time: 30 mins

Total Time: 50 mins

Servings: 16

Ingredients

• 8 cups chicken broth

• ½ cup fresh lemon juice

• ½ cup shredded carrots

• ½ cup finely chopped onion

• ½ cup finely chopped celery

• 6 tablespoons chicken soup base

• ¼ teaspoon ground white pepper

• ¼ cup margarine

• ¼ cup all-purpose flour

• 8 egg yolks

• 1 cup cooked white rice

• 1 cup diced, cooked chicken meat

• 16 slices lemon

Directions

1. Combine chicken broth, lemon juice, carrots, onions, celery, soup base, and white pepper in a large pot. Bring to a boil over high heat, then reduce heat and simmer for 15 to 20 minutes, or until the vegetables are tender.

2. Blend margarine and flour in a small bowl; gradually stir into soup mixture. Simmer, stirring frequently, for 8 to 10 minutes.

3. Meanwhile, beat egg yolks in a bowl until light in color. Gradually whisk in some hot soup, using a ladle to pour in a thin stream while whisking the egg yolks vigorously. Add egg mixture to the pot in same manner, and heat through.

4. Add rice and chicken; cook until warmed through. Ladle hot soup into bowls and garnish with lemon slices.

Recipe Tip

If the chicken broth you are using is already well seasoned, you may not need to add additional chicken base. We recommend tasting the soup after Step 1 and adding chicken base to taste if needed.

Nutrition Facts (per serving)

124 Calories

7g Fat

9g Carbs

8g Protein

Shmunky's Colby Jack Cheddar Biscuits

These biscuits have an amazing aroma and taste that will turn any grump into a jolly lad! They are crispy on the outside, yet soft and puffy in the center. They freeze well too, for making large batches. This recipe is best when handmade, so try not to be tempted by your mixers.

Prep Time: 15 mins

Cook Time: 20 mins

Total Time: 35 mins

Servings: 8

Yield: 16 biscuits

Ingredients

- 1 teaspoon olive oil

- 2 cups all-purpose flour

- 1 tablespoon baking powder

- 1 ½ teaspoons dried parsley

- ⅛ teaspoon ground thyme

- 1 teaspoon salt

- 1 teaspoon white sugar

- 1 cup shredded Colby-Monterey Jack cheese

- ¼ cup shredded white Cheddar cheese

- 6 tablespoons butter

- 1 cup 2% milk

Directions

1. Preheat oven to 400 degrees F (200 degrees C). Using olive oil, grease a baking sheet.

2. With a fork, mix together the flour, baking powder, parsley, thyme, salt, sugar, Colby-Monterey Jack cheese, and white Cheddar cheese together in a bowl. Cut the butter into the flour mixture in coarse chunks, then use the fork to further cut the butter into the flour-cheese mixture until the mixture resembles coarse crumbs. Lightly stir in the milk just until the dough holds together.

3. Drop the batter by heaping 1/8-cup measuring cup onto the prepared baking sheet, and bake in the preheated oven until risen and golden brown, 20 to 30 minutes.

Cook's Notes

Baking times vary depending on your type of oven and elevation. I suggest you start watching the biscuits around 12 minutes into baking time and checking on them every 5 minutes after that.

Nutrition Facts (per serving)

293 Calories

17g Fat

27g Carbs

9g Protein

Tzatziki Sauce (Yogurt and Cucumber Dip)

Drain some low-fat yogurt overnight to make this yummy cucumber dressing. This is a delicious topping for grilled chicken or meat. It's also a great dip for veggies and pita chips.

Prep Time: 25 mins

Additional Time: 10 hrs

Total Time: 10 hrs 25 mins

Servings: 16

Yield: 2 cups

Ingredients

• 1 (16 ounce) container low-fat plain yogurt

• 1 cucumber, peeled, seeded, and grated

• 1 clove garlic, minced

- 1 tablespoon chopped fresh parsley

- 1 tablespoon chopped fresh mint

- 1 tablespoon fresh lemon juice

- salt and pepper to taste

Directions

1. Line a colander with two layers of cheesecloth and place it over a medium bowl. Place the yogurt on the cheesecloth and cover the colander with plastic wrap. Allow yogurt to drain overnight.

2. Lay grated cucumber on a plate lined with paper towel; allow to drain 1 to 2 hours.

3. Combine the drained yogurt, cucumber, garlic, parsley, mint, lemon juice, salt, and pepper in a bowl. Refrigerate for at least 2 hours before serving.

Nutrition Facts (per serving)

21 Calories

1g Fat

3g Carbs

2g Protein

Savory Roasted Root Vegetables

Prep Time: 30 mins

Cook Time: 45 mins

Total Time: 1 hr 15 mins

Servings: 6

Yield: 6 servings

Ingredients

• 1 cup diced, raw beet

• 4 carrots, diced

• 1 onion, diced

• 2 cups diced potatoes

• 4 cloves garlic, minced

• ¼ cup canned garbanzo beans (chickpeas), drained

• 2 tablespoons olive oil

- 1 tablespoon dried thyme leaves

- salt and pepper to taste

- ⅓ cup dry white wine

- 1 cup torn beet greens

Directions

1. Preheat an oven to 400 degrees F (200 degrees C).

2. Place the beet, carrot, onion, potatoes, garlic, and garbanzo beans into a 9x13 inch baking dish. Drizzle with the olive oil, then season with thyme, salt, and pepper. Mix well.

3. Bake, uncovered, in the preheated oven for 30 minutes, stirring once midway through baking. Remove the baking dish from the oven, and stir in the wine. Return to the oven, and bake until the wine has mostly evaporated and the vegetables are tender, about 15 minutes more. Stir in the beet greens, allowing them to wilt from the heat of the vegetables. Season to taste with salt and pepper before serving.

Nutrition Facts (per serving)

143 Calories

5g Fat

21g Carbs

3g Protein

Seasoned Roasted Root Vegetables

Prep Time: 30 mins

Cook Time: 45 mins

Total Time: 1 hr 15 mins

Servings: 10

Ingredients

• olive oil cooking spray

• 1 butternut squash - peeled, seeded, and cut into 1-inch pieces

• 1 large sweet potato, peeled and cut into 1-inch cubes

• 1 (10 ounce) package frozen Brussels sprouts, thawed and halved

• 1 onion, halved and thickly sliced

• 1 parsnip, peeled and sliced

• 3 carrots, cut into large chunks

• 2 tablespoons olive oil, or as needed

• 1 teaspoon ground thyme

• 1 teaspoon dried rosemary

• 1 pinch salt

• ground black pepper to taste

Directions

1. Preheat the oven to 400 degrees F (200 degrees C). Spray a baking sheet with cooking spray.

2. Combine butternut squash, sweet potato, Brussels sprouts, onion, parsnip, and carrots in a large bowl. Drizzle with olive oil and toss to coat. Add thyme, rosemary, salt, and black pepper; toss again. Transfer coated vegetables to the prepared baking sheet.

3. Roast vegetables in the preheated oven for 25 minutes; stir and continue roasting until vegetables are slightly brown and tender, about 20 more minutes.

Nutrition Facts (per serving)

149 Calories

3g Fat

30g Carbs

3g Protein

Taste of India Roasted Root Vegetables

Prep Time: 30 mins

Cook Time: 40 mins

Total Time: 1 hr 10 mins

Servings: 6

Yield: 6 servings

Ingredients

- 1 medium red onion, cut into 8 wedges
- 3 carrots, peeled and chopped into 1-inch pieces
- 3 parsnips, peeled and cut into 1-inch chunks
- 3 medium beets, peeled and cut into 1/2-inch cubes

- 1 medium sweet potatoes, peeled and cut into 1-inch pieces
- 4 tablespoons extra-virgin olive oil
- 1 teaspoon ground ginger
- 1 teaspoon ground coriander
- 1 teaspoon ground cumin
- ½ teaspoon ground turmeric
- ¼ teaspoon garlic powder
- ¼ teaspoon cayenne pepper, or to taste (Optional)
- 1 pinch salt and freshly ground black pepper to taste
- 2 tablespoons chopped fresh cilantro (Optional)

Directions

1. Preheat the oven to 425 degrees F (220 degrees C). Line a baking sheet with parchment paper.
2. Combine red onion, carrots, parsnips, beets, and sweet potato in a large bowl. Toss vegetables with olive oil.
3. Combine ginger, coriander, cumin, turmeric, garlic, cayenne, salt, and pepper in a small bowl.

Sprinkle spice mix over the vegetables and toss to coat evenly. Spread vegetables out evenly on the prepared baking sheet.

4. Roast on the center rack of the preheated oven until beet pieces can easily be pierced with a fork, about 40 minutes.
5. Garnish with fresh cilantro. Serve warm or at room temperature.

Cook's Note:

If not using parchment paper, grease the pan well with additional extra-virgin olive oil. If the vegetables appear to be drying out during the roasting time, use a sprayer to mist with additional extra virgin olive oil.

Nutrition Facts (per serving)

210 Calories

10g Fat

30g carbs

3g Protein

Creamy Roasted Parsnip Soup

Prep Time: 30 mins

Cook Time: 50 mins

Total Time: 1 hr 20 mins

Servings: 10

Yield: 10 cups

Ingredients

• 2 pounds parsnips, peeled and cut into 1/2 inch pieces

• 3 carrots, peeled and cut into 1/2-inch pieces

• 2 tablespoons olive oil, divided

• sea salt and ground black pepper to taste

• 1 large onion, diced

• 3 stalks celery, diced

• 1 tablespoon butter

• 1 tablespoon brown sugar

• 3 cloves garlic, minced

• 1 teaspoon ground ginger

• ½ teaspoon ground cardamom

• ½ teaspoon ground allspice

• ½ teaspoon ground nutmeg

• ¼ teaspoon cayenne pepper

• 4 cups chicken stock

• 1 cup whole milk

• ½ cup heavy cream

Directions

1. Preheat the oven to 425 degrees F (220 degrees C).

2. Place parsnips and carrots in a mixing bowl; sprinkle with 1 tablespoon olive oil and toss to coat. Season with salt and pepper. Spread vegetables evenly onto a baking sheet.

3. Roast in the preheated oven until vegetables are tender and parsnips are golden brown, about 30 minutes.

4. Heat remaining 1 tablespoon olive oil in a large saucepan over medium heat. Cook and stir onion and celery in hot oil until softened and onion is beginning to turn golden brown, about 5 minutes. Reduce heat to low; stir in butter, brown sugar, garlic, and roasted parsnips and carrots. Continue to cook and stir until vegetables are very soft and beginning to brown, about 5 to 10 minutes.

5. Season with ginger, cardamom, allspice, nutmeg, and cayenne pepper; stir for 1 minute. Pour in chicken stock; bring to a boil over medium-high heat. Reduce heat to medium-low, partially cover, and simmer gently for 5 to 10 minutes.

6. Working in batches, pour soup into a blender, filling the pitcher no more than halfway full. Hold down the lid of the blender with a folded kitchen towel and carefully start the blender, using a few quick pulses to get soup moving before leaving it on to purée. Pour blended soup into a clean pot.

7. Stir in milk and cream. Return to a simmer over medium-low heat. Season with salt and pepper to serve.

Recipe Tip

You can also use a stick blender to purée the soup right in the cooking pot.

Nutrition Facts (per serving)

187 Calories

10g Fat

24g Carbs

3g Protein

Cream of Asparagus Soup

This easy creamy asparagus soup is perfect for making the most of fresh asparagus when it's in season — take advantage!

Prep Time: 15 mins

Cook Time: 25 mins

Total Time: 40 mins

Servings: 4

Ingredients

• 1 pound fresh asparagus, trimmed and cut into 1-inch pieces

• 1 (14.5 ounce) can chicken broth, divided

• ½ cup chopped onion

• 2 tablespoons butter

• 2 tablespoons all-purpose flour

• 1 teaspoon salt, or to taste

• 1 pinch ground black pepper

• 1 cup milk

• ½ cup sour cream

• 1 teaspoon fresh lemon juice

Directions

1. Combine asparagus, 1/2 cup chicken broth, and onion in a large saucepan; cover and bring to a boil over high heat. Reduce heat to medium-low and simmer,

uncovered, until asparagus is tender, about 12 minutes. Transfer the mixture to a blender; puree until smooth and set aside.

2. In the same saucepan, melt butter over medium-low heat. Stir in flour, salt, and pepper; cook, stirring constantly, for 2 minutes.

3. Increase heat to medium; add remaining chicken broth, stirring constantly, until the mixture boils. Stir in pureed asparagus and milk.

4. Place sour cream in a small bowl and stir in a ladleful of hot soup until blended; pour into the soup and stir in lemon juice. Warm soup through to serving temperature, without boiling. Serve immediately.

Nutrition Facts (per serving)

197 Calories

13g Fat

15g Carbs

7g Protein

This asparagus risotto is flavored with garlic, white wine, lemon, and Parmesan cheese. I like to serve this as a main dish under some steamed halibut or other white fish.

Prep Time: 9 mins

Cook Time: 35 mins

Total Time: 44 mins

Servings: 4

Ingredients

• 20 fresh asparagus spears, trimmed

• 4 cups low-sodium chicken broth

• 2 tablespoons olive oil

• 1 small onion, diced

• 1 stalk celery, diced

• ¼ teaspoon salt

• ¼ teaspoon ground black pepper

- 1 cup Arborio rice

- 1 clove garlic, minced

- ½ cup dry white wine

- ¼ cup freshly grated Parmesan cheese

- 2 tablespoons lemon juice

- ½ teaspoon lemon zest

Directions

1. Place a steamer insert into a saucepan and fill with water to just below the bottom of the steamer. Bring water to a boil. Add asparagus, cover, and steam until tender, about 5 minutes. Cut asparagus into 1-inch pieces; set aside.

2. Meanwhile, heat chicken broth in a saucepan over medium heat; keep at a simmer while preparing risotto.

3. Heat olive oil in a large skillet over medium heat. Add onion and celery; cook and stir until vegetables are tender, about 5 minutes. Season with salt and black

pepper. Stir in Arborio rice and garlic; cook and stir until rice is lightly toasted, about 5 more minutes.

4. Stir in white wine and simmer until it has mostly evaporated, then stir in 1/3 of the hot chicken broth; continue stirring until rice has absorbed liquid and turned creamy. Repeat this process twice more, stirring constantly. Stirring in the broth should take 15 to 20 minutes in all. When finished, rice should be tender yet firm to the bite. Stir in asparagus.

5. Remove from heat and mix in Parmesan cheese, lemon juice, and lemon zest. Serve immediately.

Nutrition Facts (per serving)

357 Calories

9g Fat

53g Carbs

11g Protein

Broccoli Risotto

A rich and creamy broccoli risotto with just a hint of lemon.

Prep Time: 15 mins

Cook Time: 35 mins

Total Time: 50 mins

Servings: 6

Ingredients

• 2 tablespoons olive oil

• 3 tablespoons butter

• ½ large sweet onion, finely chopped

• 4 cloves garlic, chopped

• 1 ½ cups Arborio rice

• ½ cup dry white wine (such as Sauvignon Blanc)

• 2 tablespoons lemon juice

• 5 cups hot chicken broth

- 1 cup heavy cream

- 3 cups cooked broccoli florets

- 2 tablespoons chopped fresh chives

- 1 tablespoon grated Parmesan cheese

- 1 ½ tablespoons grated Asiago cheese

- salt and pepper to taste

Directions

1. Heat olive oil and butter in a large, heavy-bottomed saucepan over medium-high heat. Add onion and garlic; cook and stir until onion begins to turn golden brown at the edges, about 2 minutes.

2. Pour in rice, and stir until rice is coated in oil and has started to toast, 3 to 4 minutes. Reduce heat to medium and stir in white wine and lemon juice. Cook and stir until wine has mostly evaporated, then stir in 1/3 of the chicken broth; continue stirring until incorporated.

3. Repeat this process twice more, stirring constantly. Stirring in broth should take 15 to 20 minutes in all. Stir

in cream and cook 5 minutes before stirring in broccoli, chives, Parmesan cheese, and Asiago cheese. Cook and stir until risotto is hot; season to taste with salt and pepper before serving.

Nutrition Facts (per serving)

482 Calories

26g Fat

53g Carbs

7g Protein

Gourmet Mushroom Risotto

Prep Time: 20 mins

Cook Time: 25 mins

Total Time: 45 mins

Servings: 6

Ingredients

• 6 cups chicken broth, or as needed

• 3 tablespoons olive oil, divided

- 1 pound portobello mushrooms, thinly sliced

- 1 pound white mushrooms, thinly sliced

- 2 medium shallots, diced

- 1 ½ cups Arborio rice

- ½ cup dry white wine

- 4 tablespoons butter

- 3 tablespoons finely chopped chives

- ⅓ cup freshly grated Parmesan cheese

- sea salt and freshly ground black pepper to taste

Directions

1. Gather all ingredients.

2. Warm broth in a saucepan over low heat.

3. Meanwhile, warm 2 tablespoons olive oil in a large saucepan over medium-high heat. Add portobello and white mushrooms; cook and stir until soft, about 3 minutes. Remove mushrooms and their liquid to a bowl; set aside.

4. Add remaining 1 tablespoon olive oil to the saucepan. Stir in shallots and cook for 1 minute. Add rice; cook and stir until rice is coated with oil and pale, golden in color, about 2 minutes.

5. Pour in wine, stirring constantly until wine is fully absorbed. Add 1/2 cup warm broth to the rice, and stir until the broth is absorbed.

6. Continue adding broth, 1/2 cup at a time, stirring constantly, until the liquid is absorbed and the rice is tender, yet firm to the bite, about 15 to 20 minutes.

7. Remove from heat. Stir in reserved mushrooms and their liquid, butter, chives, and Parmesan cheese.

8. Season with salt and pepper and serve immediately.

Nutrition Facts (per serving)

431 Calories

17g Fat

57g Carbs

11g Protein

This seafood risotto is easy to make and quicker than a classic risotto. It has a gorgeous creamy texture and taste and makes a delicious spring or summer dish!

Prep Time: 30 mins

Cook Time: 25 mins

Total Time: 55 mins

Servings: 6

Ingredients

• 2 tablespoons olive oil

• 1 large leek, cleaned and thinly sliced

• 2 cloves garlic, minced

• 1 cup Arborio rice

• 2 cups low-sodium chicken broth, divided

• 1 cup dry white wine

• ½ pound bay scallops

• ½ pound medium shrimp, peeled and deveined

- 1 cup fresh snow peas, trimmed and halved crosswise

- 1 medium red bell pepper, diced

- 3 tablespoons grated Parmesan cheese

- 2 teaspoons dried basil

- 2 tablespoons lemon juice

- ground black pepper to taste

Directions

1. Heat olive oil in a large, heavy-bottomed saucepan over medium-low heat. Add leek and garlic; cook and stir until soft, about 5 minutes. Add rice and cook for 5 minutes more, stirring frequently.

2. Pour in 1 1/2 cups chicken broth and bring to a boil over high heat, stirring occasionally. Reduce heat to medium-low and simmer, uncovered, for 5 minutes, continuing to stir occasionally. Pour in remaining chicken broth and wine; increase heat to medium and cook for about 5 more minutes, stirring constantly.

3. Add scallops, shrimp, peas, and red pepper. Cook, stirring constantly, until remaining liquid is almost absorbed and seafood has cooked, about 5 minutes. When rice is just tender and slightly creamy, season with Parmesan cheese, basil, lemon juice, and pepper.

Nutrition Facts (per serving)

330 Calories

7g Fat

40g Carbs

20g Protein

Quinoa Pudding

Prep Time: 5 mins

Cook Time: 30 mins

Total Time: 35 mins

Servings: 4

Yield: 4 servings

Ingredients

- 1 ½ cups water

- ¾ cup quinoa

- 2 cups whole milk

- 2 ripe bananas

- 2 tablespoons white sugar

- salt to taste

- ½ tablespoon butter

- ½ teaspoon vanilla extract

Directions

1. Rinse and drain the quinoa. Bring water and quinoa to a boil in a saucepan over high heat, stirring occasionally. Reduce heat, cover, and simmer for 15 minutes. Remove from the heat.

2. Blend together the milk, bananas, sugar, and salt in the bowl of a blender or food processor until smooth. Pour the milk mixture into the saucepan with the quinoa.

3. Place the pan over medium heat. Cook and stir until the mixture becomes thick and creamy, 5 to 10 minutes. Remove from the heat. Stir in the butter and vanilla and serve warm.

Nutrition Facts (per serving)

269 Calories

6g Fat

46g Carbs

9g Protein

Meringue-Topped Banana Pudding

The meringue in this meringue-topped banana pudding is stabilized by acidic cream of tartar, helping it hold its shape for decorative swoops and swirls. Avoid using a copper bowl, which reacts with acid and may discolor your meringue.

Prep Time: 20 mins

Cook Time: 10 mins

Chill Time: 2 hrs

Total Time: 2 hrs 30 mins

Servings: 8

Ingredients

• 9 ounces vanilla wafer cookies (about 65 cookies)

• 6 bananas, peeled and sliced

• 1/3 cup packed brown sugar

• 1 tablespoon cornstarch

• 1/8 teaspoon salt

• 3 large egg yolks

• 2 teaspoons vanilla extract, divided

• 2 cups whole milk or half and half

• 4 large egg whites

• 1/2 teaspoon cream of tartar

• 1/2 cup white sugar

Directions

1. Line bottom of a 2-quart baking dish with half of the cookies. Top with half of the banana slices. Repeat layers.

2. Stir together brown sugar, cornstarch, and salt in a medium saucepan until no lumps remain. Stir in egg yolks and 1 teaspoon vanilla. Set pot over medium heat and gradually stir in milk, stirring constantly, until mixture becomes thick enough to coat the back of a metal spoon, 8 to 10 minutes. Remove from heat. Let cool 1 minute. Pour milk mixture evenly over bananas and cookies. Chill, covered, at least 2 hours or up to 12 hours.

3. Mix egg whites, cream of tartar, and remaining 1 teaspoon vanilla in a medium bowl with an electric mixer until soft peaks form. With mixer running, gradually add white sugar until stiff peaks form. Spread meringue over pudding.

4. Brown top of meringue with a kitchen torch, 2 to 3 minutes. (To store, insert toothpicks into meringue

halfway up toothpick; loosely drape plastic wrap over toothpicks to cover. Chill up to 24 hours.)

Nutrition Facts (per serving)

371 Calories

9g Fat

66g Carbs

8g Protein

Pennsylvania-Dutch Pickled Beets and Eggs

Prep Time: 15 mins

Cook Time: 30 mins

Additional Time: 2 days

Total Time: 2 days 45 mins

Servings: 8

Ingredients

• 8 large eggs

• 2 (15-ounce) cans whole pickled beets, juice reserved

- 1 small onion, chopped

- 1 cup white sugar

- ¾ cup cider vinegar

- 12 whole cloves

- 2 bay leaves

- ½ teaspoon salt

- 1 pinch ground black pepper

Directions

1. Place eggs in a saucepan and cover with water. Bring to a boil, remove from heat, and let eggs stand in hot water for 15 minutes. Remove eggs from hot water, cool under cold running water, and peel.

2. Place eggs, beets, and onion in a non-reactive glass or plastic container. Set aside.

3. Combine sugar, 1 cup reserved beet juice, vinegar, cloves, bay leaves, salt, and pepper in a medium-size, non-reactive saucepan. Bring to a boil, reduce heat, and simmer for 5 minutes.

4. Pour hot liquid over eggs, beets, and onion. Cover and refrigerate 48 hours before using.

Nutrition Facts (per serving)

252 Calories

5g Fat

45g Carbs

7g Protein

Stir-Fry Chicken and Vegetables

Prep Time: 20 mins

Cook Time: 20 mins

Total Time: 40 mins

Servings: 2

Ingredients

• 6 ounces skinless, boneless chicken breast, cut into small pieces

• 2 tablespoons soy sauce

• 2 tablespoons dry sherry

- 1 tablespoon cornstarch

- 1 tablespoon vegetable oil

- 1 zucchini, cut into rounds and quartered

- 1 large green bell pepper, cut into squares

- 1 cup broccoli florets, cut into pieces

- 3 cloves garlic, minced

- ½ cup chicken broth

- 1 tablespoon vegetable oil

- 6 green onions, chopped

Directions

1. Mix chicken, soy sauce, sherry, and cornstarch together in a large bowl.

2. Heat 1 tablespoon vegetable oil in a large skillet or wok over medium-high heat; cook and stir zucchini, bell pepper, broccoli, and garlic for 2 to 3 minutes. Add chicken broth, cover, and simmer until vegetables are

tender, 4 to 5 minutes. Transfer vegetables and sauce to a large bowl and wipe the skillet clean.

3. Heat remaining 1 tablespoon vegetable oil over medium-high heat; cook and stir chicken until meat is no longer pink in the center, about 5 minutes. Stir in vegetables; continue to cook and stir for 2 to 3 minutes more. Sprinkle with green onions.

Nutrition Facts (per serving)

314 Calories

16g Fat

20g Carbs

22g Protein

Apple Banana Smoothie

Prep Time: 5 mins

Total Time: 5 mins

Servings: 2

Ingredients

- 1 medium Gala apple, peeled, cored and chopped

- 1 frozen banana, peeled and chopped

- ½ cup orange juice

- ¼ cup milk

Directions

1. Gather all ingredients.

2. Combine apple, frozen banana, orange juice, and milk in a blender; blend until smooth.

3. Pour into glasses to serve. Enjoy!

Nutrition Facts (per serving)

145 Calories

1g Fat

33g Carbs

2g Protein

CONCLUSION

Diet is an important part of the quality of life. How, when, where and with whom you share meals is a part of life that can be associated with comfort and companionship. This is also worth taking into consideration when deciding to try the SCD. It is a dietary protocol that restricts specific types of carbohydrates, such as grains and tubers, and prioritizes foods that promote gut health. Some research suggests that the SCD may help improve symptoms and disease markers in people with inflammatory bowel disease and may help some people attain remission. However, the diet is very restrictive and may be hard to follow, especially long-term. If you're interested in following the SCD, it's recommended to work with a healthcare provider who has extensive knowledge of the SCD to ensure you're following the diet in a safe and appropriate way.

www.ingramcontent.com/pod-product-compliance
Lightning Source LLC
Chambersburg PA
CBHW061924270726

48659CB00002BA/621